MAKING BABIES WHEN GETTING PREGNANT GETS HARD

Natural Approach to Improve Your Fertility, Balance Your Hormones, Get Pregnant Naturally, Prevent Miscarriage, and Improve your chance to Conceive

Important!

Making babies when Getting Pregnant Gets Hard is only for your personal use. You may not give away or include it to any product or membership site.

©2019 Bob Marsh

All Rights Reserved

No part of this eBook may be reproduced or transmitted in any form whatsoever, electronic or mechanical, including photocopying, recording, or by any informational storage or retrieval system without expressed written, dated and signed permission from the author.

Disclaimer and Legal Notices

The information presented in this book represents the views of the author as of the date of publication. Due to the rate at which conditions change, the author reserves the rights to alter and update his opinions based on the new conditions.

This book is intended for educational purposes only; it should not take the place of advice or recommendations from your healthcare provider, if you have questions about what you heard please consult your doctor.

The author does not accept any responsibilities for any liabilities resulting from the use of this information.

Results will vary for different efforts and different people.

While every attempt has been made to verify the information provided herein, the author cannot assume any responsibility for errors, inaccuracies or omissions.

Any slights of people or organizations are unintentional.

TABLE OF CONTENTS

UNDERSTANDING THE EGG QUALITY

SIGNS OF INFERTILITY IN MEN AND WOMEN

SIGNS OF INFERTILITY IN MEN

SYMPTOMS OF OVULATION

HOW TO RESTORE OVULATION

HOW TO CLEANSE YOUR UTERUS WHEN PREPARING FOR CONCEPTION

RECIPE THAT HELPS INCREASE FERTILITY

HOW TO BOOST YOUR FERTILITY

THIS IS FOR TTC (TRYING TO CONCEIVE)

RECEIPE TO TREAT INFECTION AND TTC (TRYING TO CONCEIVE)

UNDERSTANDING THE EGG QUALITY

In this book we will be looking at the sort of problems that can lead to decrease in fertility, which includes:

- ❖ Ovulation Problems
- ❖ Uterus Problem
- ❖ Age-related Problem,
- ❖ Fallopian tubes Problems which is where the egg and sperm engage

We have different tests being carried out in order to discover what the major problem is.

The typical first-line initial tests of a woman undergoing fertility evaluation include:

Hormone levels which is use to evaluate your ovarian function and thyroid, also a test to check the tubes to make sure the fallopian tubes are open

We also do an ultrasound scan to help evaluate the uterus.

As a woman ages, her fertility declines. A woman is born with eggs of about a million per ovary at birth, and by menopause they only have just about a thousand left.

Therefore, during her course of life, she loses a lot of eggs and as the number of eggs reduces the fertility goes down.

There is no certain age after which it's a cliff, it's a continuous decrease and particularly after

35 or 37 years of age fertility becomes more of an enigma. This is because of age, for women under 35 if they've tried for a year and haven't been able to conceive it deserves seeing a doctor.

But for women over 35, six months in terms of helping couples conceive is not a rubber-stamp, therefore individualized treatment depends majorly on the particular problem of the couple.

Therefore, we do the evaluation and then based on the evaluation we will both agree with a strategy that's reasonable from my viewpoint and acceptable from the patient's viewpoint.

Therefore, typical treatments may include but not limited to:

Taking fertility drugs to help the woman ovulate better, this may include artificial insemination. More importantly if there's a male factor involved.

For instance, if more aggressive treatment such as vitro fertilization is consider, the couple will be spending so much, because it is quite expensive.

Therefore, starting off on this process of trying to reproduce is important to do everything they can to maximize their own success and thereby not needing a service of an health care personnel by doing the following:

Avoiding caffeine, even if you are addicted to taking it, do not take more than one cup of coffee a day.

Stop the use of drugs most especially marijuana and cocaine.

Stop smoking, smoking kills eggs, it's the only thing I know that a woman can choose to do that kills eggs, decreases her fertility and brings earlier the age of menopause.

Therefore, when a couple embarks on trying to start a family, often they hear from family friends and others that they should have intercourse precisely during ovulation.

I'm a strong believer that when too much pressure is being put on couple, it causes a lot of stress, and that stress actually can decrease their fertility during such period.

Therefore in this book, i will be revealing some things that will help you along your journey to have your own kids, just make sure you read to the end, and make use of every method in this book.

If you do, you will share your own testimony soon.

Many people have asked me about the causes of poor quality of egg, because we know that the quality of the eggs tends to reduce as you go into your late 20s and early 30s including late 30s.

It becomes more terrible by the time you're in your 40s.

What I mean by quality is not necessarily the baby, but the live baby rate parade.

Therefore, the younger the egg, the better the egg quality.

That is really clear, but there is some women who are plagued by having a lot of poor quality eggs, and the only way to deal with that is doing IVF,.

I clomid, ivf protocol very mild elevation of FSH an equivalent mild elevation of LH.

If the LH isn't elevated just the way the FSH is, and in a mild way you don't get good egg quality.

If you're just stimulating with FSH and some drugs that have HCG but aren't really good HCG alternatives, then you're going to have just pure FSH stimulation and you won't get good quality eggs.

For women who are on the edge, it's really important to do what I call clomid mini IVF protocol, which involves just a very mild elevation of your FSH in your LH triggering with Lupron vitrified freezing the embryos, and then transferring them into a perfect uterine lining.

It's amazing some of these terrible cases with four or five or ten previous IVF cycles with poor quality eggs elsewhere with massive stimulation.

Well, we just do this very wild simulation to get good quality eggs and a better chance of high pregnancy rates.

But before considering IVF, I will suggest you carry out the method I'm about to reveal here.

SIGNS OF INFERTILITY IN MEN AND WOMEN

Common Signs of Infertility in Women

Pain during sex: some women experience painful sex in their entire lives so they've convinced themselves normal, but it's not.

This could be as a result of hormone issues to endometriosis or to other underlying conditions that could also be contributing to infertility.

Irregular periods: The normal cycle for women is 28 days long, and if it is also within a few days of that can also be considered as normal.

As long as a woman have a consistent cycles e.g a woman who has a 33 day cycle the first month a 31 day cycle the following month, and from there changed to 35 day cycle after the previous month, this can be classify as probably having normal periods.

But, when a woman cycles vary so greatly that she can't even begin to estimate when her period might arrive, such individual can be said to be experiencing irregular periods, which can be as a result of hormone issues or polycystic ovarian syndrome PCOS.

Both of these can contribute to infertility as well as painful or heavy period.

Cramps during periods as also been recorded as one of the things such people experience.

But when you experience a painful periods that interfere with your daily life may be a symptom of endometriosis c3.

Although it's not uncommon for women to have an off month, because some factors such as stress or heavy workouts can result to the temporary disappearance of your period, but if you haven't had a period in months, then you should get yourself checkup for symptoms of hormone fluctuations.

In women signs of hormone fluctuations could indicate potential issues with fertility, therefore it is important you discuss with your doctor if you experience the following:

- ❖ Skin Issues
- ❖ Thinning Hair
- ❖ Weight Gain

- ❖ Reduce Sex Drive
- ❖ Facial Hair Growth

SIGNS OF INFERTILITY IN MEN

A man's fertility, as also be noted to cause changes in sexual desire, which is linked with his hormone health changes.

In virility often governed by hormones could indicate issues with fertility to testicle pain or swelling.

We have different conditions that could lead to pain or swelling in the testicles, which many could contribute to infertility.

Small firm testicles: Testes house a man's sperm, so testicle health is paramount to male fertility.

Because small or firm testicles could indicate potential issues that should be explored by a medical practitioner.

Finding it difficult to maintain erection: The ability for a man to be able to maintain an erection is due to his hormone levels.

Reduced hormones may result into what could potentially be translate into trouble conceiving.

For issues with ejaculation similarly an inability to ejaculate is a sign that it might be time to visit a doctor.

SYMPTOMS OF OVULATION

How to know when you are ovulating

1. Water retention

2. Sensitivity in breast and tenderness

3. Cervical mucus: It is important you take note of your cervical mucus numerous times a day, because this is one of the reliable ovulation sign.

Your mucus changes in acknowledgment to being at infertile or fertile stages of your cycle.

Therefore, it is a good indicator of when your fertility has returned after having a baby.

Cervical mucus changes with variations in hormones following a period. Mucus will typically be dry, before turning sticky and then turn creamy, from there to watery form, before it's most fertile state which is clear slippery and stretchy highly fertile mucus which looks like raw white egg which is the best.

This helps the sperm on its passage to the egg so as to provide an alkaline protection from the vagina's acidic environment.

But as you get older you will have fewer days of egg with white cervical mucus(ewc M).

e.g a woman in her 20s might have up to five days of ewc M whereas , a women in her late 30s might have one or two days at most.

4. Increased libido

5. Spotting mid cycle: This is believed to be as a result of the sudden drop of estrogen, prior to ovulation which is due to there being no

progesterone right away in the lining which can cause leakage in a small amount of blood.

6. Ovulation Pain: One of the most uncomfortable ovulation sign in is ovulation pain or Middle shmear, which is a German word which means mid pain, during this period women ovulation causes a sudden regular pain in their lower abdomen.

Therefore, it is essential to understand that painful ovulation is not normal; it is only a mild sensation that is normal.

Having pain during such time could be a sign of ovarian cysts adhesions, or from previous abdominal surgery, and it could be from other health problems which are needed to be investigated right away, especially if you are trying to conceive, as pain can be a sign of a medical problem that can result into infertility.

7. Increased energy level

8. Cervical position: your cervix helps you to understand some certain things as well as when you are fertile.

Taking note of your cervix position is a helpful tool to work out when ovulation is near, you will need a few cycles to get the hang of it and understand all the variations and changes in your cervix.

The position of the cervix is best checked at the same time each day, as it doesn't remain in one spot all day.

It is necessary you wash your hands before checking your cervix.

The cervix is clever just like your cervical mucus and changes to optimize the chances of conception, when you're not fertile you will notice that your cervix will feels low, hard like the tip of your nose and dry at the same time.

To identify a fertile cervix, it will be soft more like your earlobe; high open and wet for drop in basal.

9. Heightened sense of vision smell and taste

10. Body temperature: If you want to notice a drop in your basal body temperature, it is important you chart your cycle by taking your temperature every morning upon waking, maintain same time checking every day.

Charting helps you to understand your cycle and identifying what your body is doing and what it normally does.

If you haven't been charting your cycle previously this information won't be helpful for this cycle but now is a great time to learn and start doing it.

These are specifically designed for measuring Slyder than normal fluctuations in temperature they are accurate 2 + / 0.05 degrees centigrade measuring to 2 decimal places.

We have various fertility thermometers on the market these days, but as long as it's a basal thermometer you are using, after ovulation you will notice your temperature normally rises and stays that way until your next period.

If you become pregnant your temperature stays higher this is how some women know when to expect their period, by noticing a drop in temperature around the time their period is due,

HOW TO RESTORE OVULATION

How to heal infertility using a simple and highly effective approach, we have more than 20 years of experience giving punchable the healing suggestions to hundreds of couples dealing with infertility.

We understand how much it means especially to women to get pregnant even after encountering several failures through various methods.

many couples that have failed to get success with other methods have been successful with our simple natural approach, many patients hesitate to try our Aloe Vera recipe this is because it is so simple that it is very hard to believe that it work wonders, but to be honest with you, those have followed this method with sincerity have given birth to a healthy child and also enjoy a healthy family.

I will split this into two sections

1. The female reproductive system giving importance to the mucous friction which many women ignore, because they think it is unimportant.

We strongly recommend both the husband and wife take note of this very carefully, which will help themto understand why there are problems in achieving a successful pregnancy.

Understanding the mucus pattern, the husband's problem of low sperm counts and abnormal sperm production can be overcome very easily.

2. How various fertility problems of PCOS sustain ovary irregular menstruation, miscarriages, low sperm counts and various step of abnormal **sperm production problems can be corrected through** this method **to achieve pregnancy.**

Ingredient

- ❖ Aloe Vera
- ❖ Honey

Taking one tablespoon of aloe vera juice with honey before breakfast daily for a period of 6 months is a good medicine for irregular menstruation and many female infertility problems.

Aloe Vera is set to make a woman's body fertile, we have many success stories curing many infertility problems like PCOS, irregular menstruation and other unknown causes of infertility using aloe vera and other ancient time-tested natural medicine such as black sesame seeds with palm sugar or unrefined cane sugar.

women with irregular menstruation respond very well, those with regular menstruation cycles also can take this safely for a couple of months and then discontinue it.

Women should not use this during menstruation because it increases the flow of menstrual blood.

Also women with heavy bleeding should avoid this recipe; rather they should take 3 tbsp of organically grown black sesame seeds with unrefined sugarcane.

Blend it with your blender, and take any time of the day, you can as well take it in the evening

During menstruation days pause and then stop after 6 months.

HOW TO CLEANSE YOUR UTERUS WHEN PREPARING FOR CONCEPTION

Ingredient

1 ginger

A glass cup of Hot water

Preparation

Grate the ginger and add the glass cup of hot water into it, cover and leave for 15 minutes.

After 15 minutes strain the water out using a sieve.

Usage

Serve in the morning 30 minutes before breakfast, drink on the last day of your menstrual period, just once.

Immediately you take this try as much as possible to walk around for 5 minutes.

This method is just for cleansing your uterus when preparing for conception.

RECIPE THAT HELPS INCREASE FERTILITY

The following are the ingredients you will be needing:

- ❖ 1 Fresh Banana
- ❖ Baking soda
- ❖ Milk
- ❖ 2 eggs

Note: If you don't have any medical issue this should work immediately you use this method.

This is because it's going to help increase and boost your fertility, so if your husband is medically fine you should be able to get pregnant immediately because many TTC (Trying to Conceive) who are affected with this issue have testify to this method, so try give this a trial.

Preparation

Peel the banana and cut it into different pieces, then add the baking soda, after then, break the 2 raw egg and add it to it the then blend the whole ingredients in the blender, after that add the milk to it, and you will have a creamy result. The taste is amazing.

Usage

Drink everything at once.

You should drink it 3 times in a month, during your ovulation, a day to your menstruation and after your menstruation.

If you can do this, you will achieve a great result.

Many people have testified to this method, so therefore, it will be great if you give it a trial. Just make sure that you or your spouse isn't battling with any infection, if you are it will be better if you get that treated before taking this recipe.

HOW TO BOOST YOUR FERTILITY

Here, I will let you how to get started, what you need to focus on while you're doing it, and some resources for you to get started and know what to make.

This has been write to help people to jumpstart their fertility diet, so this is a great way to start to help the body to transition towards fertility.

One of the things I found when working with people on dietary changes is that it can be somehow difficult for some people because they're not naturally attracted to the types of foods such as: fruits, vegetables even water.

We have people who do not like the taste of water.

Therefore, what i came across is that when you add things instead of focusing on taking, or focusing on don't eat this, take this out, can be a whole lot of problem for some people. In order to solve this problem, we focus on adding things into the current diet that you are currently eating and what happens within some period of time is that your taste buds begin to change, isn't that amazing?

This is because you naturally become what you wanted to eat because your taste buds we began to change.

What we're going to cover is important, and it is really simple and so all you need is just to focus on adding the below explained things to your diet every single day.

So what are these things?

The first is going to be upon waking first thing in the morning you're going start up your day by drink one quarter cup of water.

You can also put in some lemon in it and you just drink that as soon as you wake up.

You don't have to take the whole thing at a go; you can drink it while you're getting ready for the day by taking it little by little.

Eat one dark leafy vegetable every day and this can be cooked.

For instance Swiss chard or kale or spinach these are so easy to add to your dinner meal or you can put these in your smoothie.

A lot of people like to put kale, that can work as well one tip for adding greens to your smoothies is to put them in first and put them in the bottom of the blender and then put your fruit and put everything on top of it and then you blend that and it blends out really well.

Drink one fertility smoothie every day.

E.g of a fertility smoothie

- ❖ Cherries
- ❖ Cashew Milk Or Nut Milk Of Choice
- ❖ Hemp Seeds (Optional)
- ❖ Cipro Tea Powder (Optional)
- ❖ Bananas
- ❖ Pineapple
- ❖ Greens (Optional)
- ❖ Spinach

Blend all together and drink that once a day.

What makes something a fertility smoothie those by adding a fertility friendly superfood to it, so part of this step is drink 1/4 totally smoothie day that contains a fertility supportive superfood such as:

royal jelly maca which is one of my favorites greens powder

fertilia greens or spirulina

Those are all examples of a superfood that you can add to the smoothie.

I love to do my smoothies either first thing in the morning as breakfast or for lunch.

So I get that done early in the day.

So the next thing is eat one big green salad per day, this isn't like a little side salad the order at you know at a restaurant this is going to be an actual salad that's in a bowl that's larger than a cereal bowl.

Eat one big green salad per day, it's going to have lots of color in it whatever you like you can have romaine, you can have kale you can have mixed greens whatever you like is what you want to add to that salad.

THIS IS FOR TTC (TRYING TO CONCEIVE)

This recipe will help Boost fertility

Ingredients

- ❖ One Tin Liquid Milk
- ❖ Two raw Egg
- ❖ Two Pieces of Banana
- ❖ One Teaspoon of Bicarbonate Soda

Preparation

Peel the back of the banana away and then blend the two pieces of banana together.

Once done, add all the other ingredients: Milk, raw egg, bicarbonate soda and blend well.

Usage

Drink immediately after your menstrual cycle, drink it only once and on an empty stomach early in the morning, a day after you finish your menstruation.

After using this recipe, have sex with your husband more importantly during your ovulation period...

Other Benefits

This recipe also helps to regulate the menstrual cycle and ovulation, regulate hormones, prevent certain types of miscarriage, thicken the uterine lining, and improve overall health.

RECEIPE TO TREAT INFECTION AND TTC (TRYING TO CONCEIVE)

Ingredients:

- ❖ Clove 2 tablespoon
- ❖ Negro pepper 2-4
- ❖ Lime 5
- ❖ Ginger 10 pieces
- ❖ Garlic 20 pieces
- ❖ 75cl of Water
- ❖ Turmeric 8 pieces

PREPARATION:

Wash and dice the ingredients, after that, boil all the ingredients together for about 20 minutes.

For women, use this recipe during your period.

For Men, you can take it any time you like

Sieve before drinking,

Usage

Drink just a quarter of glass morning and night for 5 days

You can warm it each day before drinking.

Stop using on the 5th day

Note: Please do not take this during preg

THANK YOU!!!

OTHER AVAILABLE BOOK

The Surprising and Shocking Secret of Birthdays: Your Complete Guide to Uncover the Details about Your Life Direction, Talents, Destiny, Character, Finances, and Relationships

The Essential Guide to Stopping Kidney Disease: All-natural effective method to heal kidney disease, manage, slow or stop the progression of incurable kidney disease and improve kidney function

Recipes for Liver Rescue: How I Reversed Fatty Liver, Weight Loss Issues, Fatigue, Gallstones Quickly and Permanently When Doctors Predicted I Would Die

Heart disease solution: The Essential Guide to Beat, Prevent and Recover from Heart Attack, and all forms of Heart Disease

Made in the USA
Monee, IL
15 July 2022

99792350R00031